CONTENTS

INTRODUCTION

Cooking your food using all-natural methods is becoming a trendy revival these days. Gone are the days when people would want to cook their food using their microwave ovens. And with people finding more time to experiment in the kitchen, many try cooking methods that they would not normally use such as grilling and smoking. Many people experiment on these cooking methods not only because they have a lot of time to do kitchen experiments in their homes but the closure of their favorite restaurants meant that they are no longer able to enjoy their favorite restaurant-quality barbecue and smoked meats. So instead of just dreaming of the day when you can finally eat restaurant-caliber smoked barbecue, now is the time for you to go and get yourself a grill particularly the Traeger Grill. And let this book serve as your ultimate guide to using your Traeger Grill and cooking sumptuous grilled foods cooked at the comfort of your home.

WHAT IS THE TRAEGER GRILL?

With so many grills that are available in the market, the Traeger Grill is considered as one of the top-of-the-line grills that you can ever invest for your outdoor kitchen. This innovative grill allows you to cook authentic grilled foods yet you don't deviate with the tradition of cooking using wood pellets so you don't get that distasteful aftertaste you get from cooking in a gas grill.

Made by an Oregon-based company, the Traeger Grill has been around for many decades. This type of smoker grill is known to cook food using all-nature wood pellets so that foods do not only smell and taste great but also healthy. But unlike traditional smokers, the Traeger Grill has been innovated to provide convenience even to grill and barbecue neophytes. It comes with a motor that turns the auger thereby consistently feeding the burn pot so you can achieve even cooking.

The Advantages of Traeger Grill

The Traeger Grill is not only limited to, well, grilling. It is an essential outdoor kitchen appliance as it allows you to also bake, roast, smoke, braise, and barbecue. But more than it being a useful kitchen appliance, below are the advantages of getting your very own Traeger Grill:

- **Better flavor:** The Traeger Grill uses all-natural wood, so food comes out better-tasting compared to when you cook them in a gas or charcoal grill. In fact, there are 14 different flavors that you can impart to your food and this book will have its own chapter dedicated to those 14 flavors of pellets.

- **No flare-ups:** No flare-ups mean that food is cooked evenly on all sides. This is made possible by using indirect heat. And because there are no flare-ups, you can smoke, bake, and rose without some areas or sides of your food burning.

- **Mechanical parts are well designed and protected:** The mechanical parts of the Traeger Grill are protected particularly from fats and drippings, so it does not get stuck over time.

- **Exceptional temperature control:** The Traeger Grill has exceptional temperature control. The thing is that all you need is to set up the heat and the grill will maintain a consistent temperature even if the weather goes bad. Moreover, having a stable temperature control allows you to cook food better and tastier minus the burnt taste.

- **Built-in Wi-Fi**: All Traeger Grills have built-in Wi-Fi so you can set them up even if you are not physically present in front of your grill. Moreover, the grill also alerts you once your food is ready. With this setting, you will be able to do other important things instead of slaving in front of your grill. Lastly, it also comes with an app that allows you to check many recipes from their website.

- **Environmentally friendly**: Perhaps the main selling point of the Traeger Grill is that it is environmentally friendly. Traeger Grill uses all-natural wood pellets, so your grill does not produce harmful chemicals when you are using it... only smoky goodness.

The thing is that the Traeger Grill is more than just your average grill. It is one of the best there is, and you will definitely get your money's worth with this grill.

Control Panel

While the Traeger Grill is designed to be innovative, operating it is no rocket science. In fact, the standard digital controller or control panel of the Traeger grill is extremely easy to understand even for someone who is a novice in the kitchen.

- **Temperature Panel:** The temperature panel indicates the temperature that you want to maintain while cooking your food. Temperature is displayed in Fahrenheit.

- **Temperature Control Knob:** The temperature knob allows you to increase or decrease the temperature in increments of 25 degrees. The temperature range is from 180oF to 375oF. The temperature control knob also comes with options such as Smoke, High Temperature, and Shut Down Cycle.

- **Timer:** The latest models of Traeger Grill also comes with a timer so that your food cooks at the proper moment. This option is also especially important as you do not need to be in front of your grill to turn it off.

- **Menu:** More advanced Traeger Grills come with a menu setting that allows you to control your grill settings. You can also update the firmware version of your grill so that you can optimize its Wi-Fi connectivity.

Unboxing Your Traeger Grill

The Traeger Grill is the best modern grill that you can use to grill foods to perfection. So, if you get one, I am fairly sure that you are excited to use it immediately. But before you start firing up your new Traeger Grill, below are some things that you need to know about unboxing your grill.

- **Work on a stable and flat surface:** Assemble the grill on a clean and flat surface so that it can stand on stable ground.

- **Attach the leg to the grill:** Flip the grill upside down and Install the legs. The grill is very heavy so you might want help while lifting it. Fasten the legs to the grill. Use bolts and nuts to fasten the two components together. Once the feet are installed properly, flip the grill so that it stands on its legs.

- **Attach the smokestack and chimney cap:** Insert the smokestack using bolts and nuts. The chimney cap should be installed once the smokestack is installed. Install the side lift handle and check for packaging inside the grill. Remove the packaging and attach the drip tray.

SEASONING YOUR GRILL FOR FIRST TIME USE

When it comes to using your new Traeger Grill, the secret is all about the seasoning. Seasoning the grill is the process of heating as well as oiling the grates to optimize your grill and remove manufacturing contaminants. Moreover, if you do not season your grill properly, you will end up eating having nasty stuff stuck on your food. The thing is that manufacturers use industrial oils and waxes to coat the surfaces of your device. Moreover, part of the manufacturing process also produces metal shavings, residual paint, and dust that may get into your food especially if you do not season your grill properly.

Why Should You Season Your Grill?

But more than remove manufacturing contaminants, why should you season your grill? Below are other reasons why you need to season your grill properly.

- **Better Flavor:** When you fire your grill, the fats, and juices of your meat falls into the grill and gets vaporized with high heat. The vaporized fats will coat the entire insides the grill. Thus, the more you season or fire up your grill, the more flavor adheres to your grill.

- **Grill Lasts Longer:** The grill lasts for a longer time if you season it as it prevents rust. If you take time to season your grill, you can expand the lifespan of your grill thus you can enjoy cooking your favorite grilled foods for a longer time.

How to Season Your Grill

Before you cook the first batch of your food in your new Traeger Grill, you need to season your grill using a one-time initial firing process. This process will get the most out of your Traeger Wood Pellet Grill.

- Place wood pellets in your auger tubes.

- Plug the grill into an outlet and turn it on.

- Add pellets into the hopper.

- Turn on the main power and turn the dial knob to Select Auger before choosing Prime Auger.

- The pellets must fall into the firepot. Once done, turn off the auger.

- Turn the temperature dial and set the temperature to 3500F.

- Press Ignite and close the lid. Run for 20 minutes before adjusting the temperature to High. Allow to run for another 30 minutes.

- Shut down the grill to finish seasoning.

The steps to seasoning your grill are extremely easy and once your grill shuts down, you are now ready to cook your first batch of food.

Other Tips in Seasoning Your Grill

While the instructions above are specific to the seasoning of Traeger Grills, there are also other workarounds and tips that you can follow for better seasoning. Below are some of the things that you can optionally do when seasoning your grill.

- **Rinse the grill grates:** Rinse the grill grates with water to remove heavy dust. You do not need to use dishwashing soap but if you do, make sure that you rinse the grate properly.

- **Wipe the insides of the grill with oil:** Use a paper towel to wipe the grates with vegetable oil. Make sure that the oil has a high smoke point so that it can withstand the high temperature used while seasoning the grill. The reason for wiping the insides with oil is to seal the grill. The oil can seep into the pores or cracks and will create a proper coating to protect the grill grate. However, make sure that you do not slather your grill with too much oil as it can start a fire.

- **Season your grill even if it is old:** Seasoning should not only be done for new grills but even for old grills. In order for your old grill to perform better, you need to season it regularly at least thrice a year. So how do you know that your grill needs seasoning? You will know when food sticks on to the grate and you see rusts forming.

USING HARDWOOD PELLETS: AN IN-DEPTH GUIDE

The Traeger Grill requires you to use all-natural wood pellets. The thing is that different kinds of wood pellets can impart different flavors on your food thus improving your gastronomic experience all the time. This section is intended as your in-depth guide on which hardwood pellets to use on your Traeger Grill.

- **Alder:** Alder wood pellets are versatile, and they add mild flavor and aroma to your food. This wood pellet also gives off a lot of smoke but does not overpower even the most delicate foods. Use it to cook chicken and fish. Surprisingly, alder pellets are also great for baked goods as it imparts a smoky yet sweet aroma to it.

- **Apple:** Apple pellets are great for cooking pork and poultry. It gives off a light fruity smoke thereby enhancing mild-flavored meats. Similar to alder pellets, it is also great for baked goods. You can make smoke-roasted apple pies with them to elevate the classic American pastry.

- **Cherry:** Cherry pellets can add hearty flavor and aroma to your dish. It is great for red meats such as beef and pork. It also imparts a cherry fragrance that improves the experience of eating your food.

- **Hickory:** A favorite wood pellet for savory barbecue, hickory pellets release an extraordinarily strong flavor, yet it complements all kinds of meats. However, if you find hickory pellets a bit strong, you can mix it with milder pellets such as apples and oak. Hickory pellets are great for pork barbecue.

- **Maple:** Maple pellets give off mild smoky aroma with a hint of sweetness. They are great for pork and turkey. Maple pellets are great for making holiday meats.

- **Mesquite:** Mesquite wood pellets are the signature wood used in making Texas BBQ. This type of wood pellet infuses your meats with a hearty and smoky flavor. The strong smoky flavor is great for recipes that call for something extra special. Mesquite is great for game meats as it masks off the gamey flavor of the meat.

- **Oak:** Oak pellets are great as far as smoke intensity is concerned. It is one of the smoke pellets that give off a light smoky aroma to food. However, it is stronger than both the apple and cherry wood pellets thus making it perfect for all types of meat dishes. But aside from meats, it is also great for smoked and grilled vegetables as well as fish.

- **Pecan:** Pecan wood pellets impart a nutty as well as a little spicy flavor into your food. It is great with poultry, pork, and beef. You can also use it to make baked goods particularly loaves of bread.

These are the wood pellets that you can use to cook different kinds of foods in your Traeger Grill. It is available on the store's website. You can mix different wood pellets or buy pre-mixed pellets to ensure that you get the right proportion of wood pellets to cook your favorite meals.

TIPS AND TRICKS TO USING YOUR TRAEGER GRILL

Your Traeger Grill is not only for making smoked meats. In fact, there are so many things that you can make out of this kitchen device. This section will provide you with helpful tips and tricks so that you can optimize your Traeger Grill. Make sure that you are making the most out of your Traeger Grill.

- **Use the reverse sear:** The reverse sear is a great and exciting way to cook steak. You can smoke your meats at low temperatures (1500F). Cook your meat low and slow (for around 1 hour) then remove the meat from the grill. Adjust the temperature knob to the highest temperature setting to add sear and more flavor to your food. If you are the kind of person who loves some charred parts on their meats, then this is the best setting for you. This will also give you the perfect medium-rare on your meat.

- **Put cold meat into the grill at a low setting:** This tip is immensely helpful especially if you are cooking large cuts of meat. The secret to cooking large cuts of meat with full flavor is to make sure that it pulls more smoke into the meat. To achieve this, make sure that you put cold meat into the grill and cook it at low temperature (1500F) as it gives a little more time for the smoke to take hold of the meat. Use this tip when cooking Tri-Tip, large brisket, and other large chunks of meats.

- **Use the upper racks of pellet grill for additional space:** You can put more food in your grill if you use the upper racks to give you extra space.

Using the extra space also decreases radiant heat coming from the grease tray so you will be able to utilize the heat more efficiently.

- **Place heat-proof water pan under a rack:** Putting a water pan with water under the rack allows long briskets to cook evenly and properly. Putting a water pan inside the grill creates steam that can help cook food. Moreover, it also allows the meat to cook in an ideal environment.

- **Use it as you would use an oven:** The Traeger Grill is not just a grill. To optimize its use, let your creativity run wild by cooking different kinds of foods in your grill. Think of it as an oven. What you can cook in an oven, you can cook in your pellet grill. To make your food more exciting, use different kinds of pellets to add more flavor to your foods.

- **Clean temperature probe regularly:** Clean the temperature probe of your grill every after use to ensure that it can effectively read the temperature properly. If you do not clean the temperature probe, the probe will be coated with fat and other drippings that may affect its ability to properly track the temperature inside your grill.

- **Preheat the grill before using it:** Before you use the grill, make sure that you preheat the grill for at least five minutes at 200°F at the most. Let the grill sit for five (5) minutes to preheat properly. However, for brand new Traeger Grill units, you can use the Advance Grilling Logic to preheat the grill to 2 minutes. Once the grill finishes preheating, you will hear a roaring noise from the main body. Once you hear the noise, close the lid to build up heat and smoke inside until you are ready to cook.

With these tips and tricks, you will definitely end up making your Traeger Grill the only outdoor kitchen appliance that you will ever need. Happy cooking.

CHICKEN RECIPES

Traeger Grill BBQ Chicken Breasts

☕ **Serves:** 4   🕐 **Cooking Time:** 30 minutes

INGREDIENTS:

- 4 whole chicken breasts, deboned
- ¼ cup olive oil
- 1 teaspoon pressed garlic
- 1 teaspoon Worcestershire sauce
- 1 teaspoon cayenne pepper powder
- ½ cup Traeger 'Que BBQ Sauce

DIRECTIONS:

1. In a bowl, combine all ingredients except for the Traeger 'Que BBQ Sauce and make sure to rub the chicken breasts until coated with the mixture. Allow to marinate in the fridge for at least overnight.
2. Place the preferred wood pellets into the Traeger Grill and fire the grill. Allow the temperature to rise to 500°F and preheat for 5 minutes. Reduce the temperature to 165°F.
3. Place the chicken on the grill grate and cook for 30 minutes.
4. Five minutes before the chicken is done, glaze the chicken with Traeger's BBQ sauce.
5. Serve immediately.

NUTRITION INFORMATION:

Calories per serving: 631; Protein: 61g; Carbs: 2.9g; Fat: 40.5g Sugar: 1.5g

Whole Smoked Chicken

Serves: 6   **Cooking Time:** 3 hours

INGREDIENTS:

- ½ cup salt
- 1 cup brown sugar
- 1 whole chicken (3 ½ pounds)
- 1 teaspoon minced garlic
- 1 lemon, halved
- 1 medium onion, quartered
- 3 whole cloves
- 5 sprigs of thyme

DIRECTIONS:

1. Dissolve the salt and sugar in 4 liters of water. Once dissolved, place the chicken in the brine and allow to marinate for 24 hours.
2. When ready to cook, fire the Traeger Grill up to 250°F and allow to preheat for 15 minutes with the lid closed. Use any wood pellet desired but we recommend using the maple wood pellet.
3. While the grill is preheating, remove the chicken from the brine and pat dry using paper towel.
4. Rub the minced garlic all over the chicken. Stuff the cavity of the chicken with the remaining ingredients.
5. Tie the legs together with a natural string.
6. Place the stuffed chicken directly on the grill grate and smoke for 3 hours until the internal temperature of the chicken is 160°F particularly in the breast part.
7. Take the chicken out and grill.

NUTRITION INFORMATION:

Calories per serving: 251; Protein: 32.6g; Carbs: 19g; Fat: 4.3g Sugar: 17.3g

Hickory Smoked Chicken Leg and Thigh Quarters

☕ **Serves:** 6   🕐 **Cooking Time:** 2 hours

INGREDIENTS:

- 6 chicken legs (with thigh and drumsticks)
- 2 tablespoons olive oil
- Traeger Poultry Rub to taste

DIRECTIONS:

1. Place all ingredients in a bowl and mix until the chicken pieces are coated in oil and rub. Allow to marinate for at least 2 hours.
2. Fire the Traeger Grill to 180°F. Close the lid and allow to preheat for 10 minutes. Use hickory wood pellets to smoke your chicken.
3. Arrange the chicken on the grill grate and smoke for one hour. Increase the temperature to 350°F and continue cooking for another hour until the chicken is golden and the juices run clean.
4. To check if the meat is cooked, insert a meat thermometer, and make sure that the temperature on the thickest part of the chicken registers at 165°F.
5. Remove the chicken and serve.

NUTRITION INFORMATION:

Calories per serving: 358 ; Protein: 50.8g; Carbs: 0g; Fat: 15.7g Sugar:0 g

Lemon Chicken Breasts

Serves: 6   **Cooking Time:** 40 minutes

INGREDIENTS:

- 1 clove of garlic, minced
- 2 teaspoons honey
- 2 teaspoons salt
- 1 teaspoon black pepper, ground
- 2 sprigs fresh thyme leaves
- 1 lemon, zested and juiced
- ½ cup olive oil
- 6 boneless chicken breasts

DIRECTIONS:

1. Make the marinade by combining the garlic, honey, salt, pepper, thyme, lemon zest, and juice in a bowl. Whisk until well-combined.
2. Place the chicken into the marinade and mix with hands to coat the meat with the marinade. Refrigerate for 4 hours.
3. When ready to grill, fire the Traeger Grill to 400°F. Close the lid and preheat for 10 minutes.
4. Drain the chicken and discard the marinade.
5. Arrange the chicken breasts directly on to the grill grate and cook for 40 minutes or until the internal temperature of the thickest part of the chicken reaches to 165°F.
6. Drizzle with more lemon juice before serving.

NUTRITION INFORMATION:

Calories per serving: 669; Protein: 60.6g; Carbs: 3g; Fat: 44.9g Sugar: 2.1g

Easy Smoked Chicken Breasts

Serves: 4   **Cooking Time:** 30 minutes

INGREDIENTS:

- 4 large chicken breasts, bones and skin removed
- 1 tablespoon olive oil
- 2 tablespoons brown sugar
- 2 tablespoons maple syrup
- 1 teaspoon celery seeds
- 2 tablespoons paprika
- 2 tablespoons salt
- 1 teaspoon black pepper
- 2 tablespoons garlic powder
- 2 tablespoons onion powder

DIRECTIONS:

1. Place all ingredients in a bowl and massage the chicken with your hands. Place in the fridge to marinate for at least 4 hours.
2. Fire the Traeger Grill to 350°F and use maple wood pellets. Close the lid and allow to preheat to 15 minutes.
3. Place the chicken on the grill a and cook for 15 minutes with the lid closed.
4. Turn the chicken over and cook for another 10 minutes.
5. Insert a thermometer into the thickest part of the chicken and make sure that the temperature reads to 165°F.
6. Remove the chicken from the grill and allow to rest for 5 minutes before slicing.

NUTRITION INFORMATION:

Calories per serving: 327 ; Protein: 40 g; Carbs: 23g; Fat: 9g Sugar: 13g

Peppered BBQ Chicken Thighs

☕ **Serves:** 6   ⊕ **Cooking Time:** 35 minutes

INGREDIENTS:

- 6 bone-in chicken thighs
- Salt and pepper to taste
- Traeger Big Game Rub to taste, optional

DIRECTIONS:

1. Place all ingredients in a bowl and allow to marinate in the fridge for at least 4 hours.
2. When ready to cook, fire the Traeger Grill to 350°F. Use apple wood pellet. Close the lid and preheat for 15 minutes.
3. Place the chicken directly on the grill grate and cook for 35 minutes. To check if the chicken is cooked thoroughly, insert a meat thermometer, and make sure that the internal temperature reads at 165°F.
4. Serve the chicken immediately.

NUTRITION INFORMATION:

Calories per serving: 430; Protein: 32g; Carbs: 1.2g; Fat: 32.1g; Sugar: 0.4g

Hickory Smoked Chicken

☕ **Serves:** 4   🕐 **Cooking Time:** 30 minutes

INGREDIENTS:

- 4 chicken breasts
- ¼ cup olive oil
- 1 teaspoon pressed garlic
- 1 tablespoon Worcestershire sauce
- Kirkland Sweet Mesquite Seasoning as needed
- 1 button Traeger Honey Bourbon Sauce

DIRECTIONS:

1. Place all ingredients in a bowl except for the Bourbon sauce. Massage the chicken until all parts are coated with the seasoning.
2. Allow to marinate in the fridge for 4 hours.
3. Once ready to cook, fire the Traeger Grill to 350ºF. Use Hickory wood pellets and close the lid. Preheat for 15 minutes.
4. Place the chicken directly into the grill grate and cook for 30 minutes. Flip the chicken halfway through the cooking time.
5. Five minutes before the cooking time ends, brush all surfaces of the chicken with the Honey Bourbon Sauce.
6. Serve immediately.

NUTRITION INFORMATION:

Calories per serving: 622; Protein: 60.5g; Carbs: 1.1g; Fat: 40.3g Sugar: 0.4g

Traeger Smoked Chicken and Potatoes

🍵 **Serves:** 4   ⊕ **Cooking Time:** 1 hour and 30 minutes

INGREDIENTS:

- 1 2.5-pounds rotisserie chicken
- 2 tablespoon coconut sugar
- 1 tablespoons onion powder
- 2 tablespoon garlic powder
- 1 teaspoon cayenne pepper powder
- 2 teaspoon kosher salt
- 4 tablespoons olive oil
- 2 pounds creamer potatoes, scrubbed and halved
- A dash of black pepper powder

DIRECTIONS:

1. Place the chicken in a bowl. In a smaller bowl, combine the coconut sugar, onion powder, garlic powder, cayenne pepper powder, and salt. Add in the olive oil. Rub the mixture into the chicken and allow to marinate for 4 hours in the fridge.
2. Fire the Traeger Grill to 400°F and close the lid. Preheat to 15 minutes.
3. Place the seasoned chicken in a heat-proof dish and place the potatoes around the chicken. Season the potatoes with salt.
4. Place in the grill and cook for 30 minutes. Lower the heat to 250°F and cook for another hour.
5. Insert a meat thermometer in the thickest part of the chicken and make sure that the temperature reads at 165°F. Flip the chicken halfway through the cooking time for even browning.

NUTRITION INFORMATION:

Calories per serving: 991; Protein: 79.7g; Carbs: 49.8g; Fat: 73.6g Sugar: 6.5g

Peach and Basil Grilled Chicken

Serves: 4   **Cooking Time:** 35 minutes

INGREDIENTS:

- 4 boneless chicken breasts
- ½ cup peach preserves, unsweetened
- ½ cup olive oil
- ¼ cup apple cider vinegar
- 3 tablespoons lemon juice
- 2 tablespoons Dijon mustard
- 1 garlic clove, crushed
- ½ teaspoon red hot sauce
- ½ cup fresh basil leaves, chopped
- Salt to taste
- 4 peaches, halved, pit removed

DIRECTIONS:

1. Place chicken in a bowl and stir in the peach preserves, olive oil, vinegar, lemon juice, Dijon mustard, garlic, red hot sauce, and basil leaves.
2. Massage the chicken until all surfaces are coated with the marinade. Marinate in the fridge for 4 hours.
3. Once ready to cook, fire the Traeger Grill to 400ºF. Use apple wood pellets. Close the lid and preheat for 15 minutes.
4. Place the chicken directly on the grill grate and cook for 35 minutes.
5. Flip the chicken halfway through the cooking time.
6. Ten minutes before the cooking time ends, place the peach halves and grill.
7. Serve with the chicken.

NUTRITION INFORMATION:

Calories per serving: 777; Protein: 61g; Carbs: 9.8g; Fat: 54.2g Sugar: 8g

Bourbon BBQ Smoked Chicken Wings

☕ **Serves:**8   ⊕ **Cooking Time:** 24 minutes

INGREDIENTS:

- 4 pounds chicken wings, patted dry
- 2 tablespoons olive oil
- Salt and pepper to taste
- ½ medium yellow onions, minced
- 5 cloves garlic, mince
- ½ cup bourbon
- 2 cups ketchup
- 1/3 cup apple cider vinegar
- 2 tablespoons liquid smoke
- ½ teaspoon kosher salt
- ½ teaspoon black pepper
- A dash of hot sauce

DIRECTIONS:

1. Place the chicken in a bowl and drizzle with olive oil. Season with salt and pepper to taste. In another bowl, combine the rest of the ingredients and set aside.
2. Fire the Traeger Grill to 400°F. Use hickory wood pellets. Close the lid and allow to preheat for 15 minutes.
3. Place the chicken on the grill grate and cook for 12 minutes on each side.
4. Using a brush, brush the chicken wings with bourbon sauce on all sides.
5. Flip the chicken and cook for another 12 minutes with the lid closed.

NUTRITION INFORMATION:

Calories per serving: 384 ; Protein: 50.7g; Carbs: 17.8 g; Fat: 11.5g Sugar: 13.1g

Smoked Chicken Thighs

Serves: 6   **Cooking Time:** 24 minutes.

INGREDIENTS:

- 6 chicken thighs
- ½ cup commercial BBQ sauce of your choice
- 1 ½ tablespoon poultry spice
- 4 tablespoons butter

DIRECTIONS:

1. Place all ingredients in a bowl except for the butter. Massage the chicken to make sure that the chicken is coated with the marinade.
2. Place in the fridge to marinate for 4 hours.
3. Fire the Traeger Grill to 350ºF. Use hickory wood pellets. Close the lid and preheat for 15 minutes.
4. When ready to cook, place the chicken on the grill grate and cook for 12 minutes on each side.
5. Before serving the chicken, brush with butter on top.

NUTRITION INFORMATION:

Calories per serving: 504; Protein: 32.4g; Carbs: 2.7g; Fat: 39.9g Sugar: 0.9g

Smoked Lemon Chicken Breasts

Serves: 6   **Cooking Time:** 30 minutes

INGREDIENTS:

- 2 lemons, zested and juiced
- 1 clove of garlic, minced
- 2 teaspoons honey
- 2 teaspoons salt
- 1 teaspoon ground black pepper
- 2 sprigs fresh thyme
- ½ cup olive oil
- 6 boneless chicken breasts

DIRECTIONS:

1. Place all ingredients in a bowl. Massage the chicken breasts so that it is coated with the marinade.
2. Place in the fridge to marinate for at least 4 hours.
3. Fire the Traeger Grill to 350ºF. Use apple wood pellets. Close the grill lid and preheat for 15 minutes.
4. Place the chicken breasts on the grill grate and cook for 15 minutes on both sides.
5. Serve immediately or drizzle with lemon juice.

NUTRITION INFORMATION:

Calories per serving: 671 ; Protein: 60.6 g; Carbs: 3.5 g; Fat: 44.9g Sugar: 2.3g

Rustic Maple Smoked Chicken Wings

Serves: 16   **Cooking Time:**

INGREDIENTS:

- 16 chicken wings
- 1 tablespoon olive oil
- 1 tablespoon Traeger Chicken Rub
- 1 cup Traeger 'Que BBQ Sauce or other commercial BBQ sauce of choice

DIRECTIONS:

1. Place all ingredients in a bowl except for the BBQ sauce. Massage the chicken breasts so that it is coated with the marinade.
2. Place in the fridge to marinate for at least 4 hours.
3. Fire the Traeger Grill to 350°F. Use maple wood pellets. Close the grill lid and preheat for 15 minutes.
4. Place the wings on the grill grate and cook for 12 minutes on each side with the lid closed.
5. Once the chicken wings are done, place in a clean bowl.
6. Pour over the BBQ sauce and toss to coat with the sauce.

NUTRITION INFORMATION:

Calories per serving: 230 ; Protein: 37.5g; Carbs: 2.2g; Fat: 7g Sugar: 1.3g

Grilled Sweet and Sour Chicken

Serves: 6   **Cooking Time:** 35 minutes

INGREDIENTS:

- 6 cups water
- 1/3 cup salt
- ¼ cup brown sugar
- ¼ cup soy sauce
- 6 chicken breasts, boneless
- 1 cup granulated white sugar
- ½ cup ketchup
- 1 cup apple cider vinegar
- 2 tablespoons soy sauce
- 1 teaspoon garlic powder

DIRECTIONS:

1. Place the water, salt, brown sugar, and soy sauce in a large bowl. Stir until well combined. Add in the chicken breasts into the brine and allow to soak for 24 hours in the refrigerator.
2. Fire the Traeger Grill to 350°F. Use maple wood pellets. Close the grill lid and preheat for 15 minutes.
3. Place the breasts on the grill grate and cook for 35 minutes on each side with the lid closed. Flip the chicken halfway through the cooking time.
4. Meanwhile, place the remaining ingredients in a bowl and stir until combined.
5. Ten minutes before the chicken breasts are cooked, brush with the sauce.
6. Serve immediately.

NUTRITION INFORMATION:

Calories per serving: 675 ; Protein: 61.9g; Carbs: 35.8g; Fat: 29.7g Sugar: 32.7g

Chile-Lime Rubbed Chicken

Serves: 6　　**Cooking Time:** 40 minutes

INGREDIENTS:

- 3 tablespoons chili powder
- 2 tablespoons extra virgin olive oil
- 2 teaspoons lime zest
- 3 tablespoons lime juice
- 1 tablespoon garlic, minced
- 1 teaspoon ground coriander
- 1 teaspoon ground black pepper
- A pinch of cinnamon
- 1 chicken, spatchcocked

- 1 teaspoon ground cumin
- 1 teaspoon dried oregano
- 1 ½ teaspoons salt

DIRECTIONS:

1. In a bowl, place the chili powder, olive oil, lime zest, juice, garlic, coriander, cumin, oregano, salt, pepper, cinnamon, and cinnamon in a bowl. Mix to form a paste.
2. Place the chicken cut-side down on a chopping board and flatten using the heel of your hand. Carefully, break the breastbone to flatten the chicken.
3. Generously rub the spices all over the chicken and make sure to massage the chicken with the spice rub. Place in a baking dish and refrigerate for 24 hours in the fridge.
4. When ready to cook, fire the Traeger Grill to 400°F. Use maple wood pellets. Close the grill lid and preheat for 15 minutes.
5. Place the chicken breastbone-side down on the grill grate and cook for 40 minutes or until a thermometer inserted in the thickest part reads at 165°F.
6. Make sure to flip the chicken halfway through the cooking time.
7. Once cooked, transfer to a plate and allow to rest before carving the chicken.

NUTRITION INFORMATION:
Calories per serving: 213; Protein: 33.1g; Carbs: 3.8g; Fat: 7g Sugar: 0.5g

Smoked Chicken with Apricot BBQ Glaze

Serves: 6   **Cooking Time:** 30 minutes

INGREDIENTS:

- 2 whole chicken, halved
- 4 tablespoon Traeger Chicken Rub
- 1 cup Trager Apricot BBQ Sauce

DIRECTIONS:

1. Massage the chicken with the chicken rub. Allow to marinate for 2 hours in the fridge.
2. When ready to cook, fire the Traeger Grill to 350ºF. Use preferred wood pellets. Close the grill lid and preheat for 15 minutes.
3. Place the chicken on the grill grate and grill for 15 minutes on each side. Baste the chicken with Apricot BBQ glaze.
4. Once cooked, allow to rest for 10 minutes before slicing.

NUTRITION INFORMATION:

Calories per serving: 304; Protein: 49g; Carbs: 10.2g; Fat: 6.5g Sugar: 8.7g

Lemon Rosemary and Beer Marinated Chicken

🍵 **Serves:** 6   ⊕ **Cooking Time:** 55 minutes

INGREDIENTS:

- 1 whole chicken
- 1 lemon, zested and juiced
- 1 teaspoon salt
- 1 teaspoon ground black pepper
- 1 teaspoon rosemary, chopped
- 12-ounce beer, apple-flavored

DIRECTIONS:

1. Place all ingredients in a bowl and allow the chicken to marinate for at least 12 hours in the fridge.
2. When ready to cook, fire the Traeger Grill to 350°F. Use preferred wood pellets. Close the grill lid and preheat for 15 minutes.
3. Place the chicken on the grill grate and cook for 55 minutes.
4. Cook until the internal temperature reads at 165°F.
5. Take the chicken out and allow to rest before carving.

NUTRITION INFORMATION:

Calories per serving: 288; Protein: 36.1g; Carbs: 4.4g; Fat: 13.1g Sugar: 0.7g

Hot and Sweet Spatchcocked Chicken

Serves:8   **Cooking Time:**55 minutes

INGREDIENTS:

- 1 whole chicken, spatchcocked
- ¼ cup Traeger Chicken Rub
- 2 tablespoons olive oil
- ½ cup Traeger Sweet and Heat BBQ Sauce

DIRECTIONS:

1. Place the chicken breastbone-side down on a flat surface and press the breastbone to break it and flatten the chicken. Sprinkle the Traeger Chicken Rub all over the chicken and massage until the bird is seasoned well. Allow the chicken to rest in the fridge for at least 12 hours.
2. When ready to cook, fire the Traeger Grill to 350°F. Use preferred wood pellets. Close the grill lid and preheat for 15 minutes.
3. Before cooking the chicken, baste with oil. Place on the grill grate and cook on both sides for 55 minutes.
4. 20 minutes before the cooking time, baste the chicken with Traeger Sweet and Heat BBQ Sauce.
5. Continue cooking until a meat thermometer inserted in the thickest part of the chicken reads at 165°F.
6. Allow to rest before carving the chicken.

NUTRITION INFORMATION:

Calories per serving: 200; Protein: 30.6g; Carbs: 1.1g; Fat: 7.4g Sugar: 0.6g

Roasted Chicken with Pimenton Potatoes

Serves: 16   **Cooking Time:** 1 hour

INGREDIENTS:

- 2 whole chicken
- 6 clove garlic, minced
- 2 tablespoons salt
- 3 tablespoons pimento (smoked paprika)
- 3 tablespoons extra virgin olive oil
- 2 bunch fresh thyme
- 3 pounds Yukon gold potatoes

DIRECTIONS:

1. Season the whole chicken with garlic, salt, paprika, olive oil, and thyme. Massage the chicken to coat all surface of the chicken with the spices. Tie the legs together with a string. Place in a baking dish and place the potatoes on the side. Season the potatoes with salt and olive oil.
2. Allow the chicken to rest in the fridge for 4 hours.
3. When ready to cook, fire the Traeger Grill to 300°F. Use preferred wood pellets. Close the grill lid and preheat for 15 minutes.
4. Place the chicken and potatoes in the grill and cook for 1 hour until a thermometer inserted in the thickest part of the chicken comes out clean.
5. Remove from the grill and allow to rest before carving.

NUTRITION INFORMATION:

Calories per serving: 210; Protein: 26.1g; Carbs: 15.3g; Fat: 4.4g Sugar: 0.7g

PORK RECIPES

Smoked Baby Back Ribs

Serves: 10 **Cooking Time:** 2 hours

INGREDIENTS:

- 3 racks baby back ribs
- Salt and pepper to taste

DIRECTIONS:

1. Clean the ribs by removing the extra membrane that covers it. Pat dry the ribs with a clean paper towel. Season the baby back ribs with salt and pepper to taste. Allow to rest in the fridge for at least 4 hours before cooking.
2. Once ready to cook, fire the Traeger Grill to 225°F. Use hickory wood pellets when cooking the ribs. Close the lid and preheat for 15 minutes.
3. Place the ribs on the grill grate and cook for two hours. Carefully flipping the ribs halfway through the cooking time for even cooking.

NUTRITION INFORMATION:

Calories per serving: 1037; Protein: 92.5g; Carbs: 1.4g; Fat: 73.7g Sugar: 0.2g

Smoked Apple Pork Tenderloin

☕ Serves: 8   🕐 **Cooking Time:** 3 hours

INGREDIENTS:

- ½ cup apple juice
- 3 tablespoons honey
- 3 tablespoons Traeger Pork and Poultry Rub
- ¼ cup brown sugar
- 2 tablespoons thyme leaves
- ½ tablespoons black pepper
- 2 pork tenderloin roasts, skin removed

DIRECTIONS:

1. In a bowl, mix together the apple juice, honey, pork and poultry rub, brown sugar, thyme, and black pepper. Whisk to mix everything.
2. Add the pork loins into the marinade and allow to soak for 3 hours in the fridge.
3. Once ready to cook, fire the Traeger Grill to 225°F. Use hickory wood pellets when cooking the ribs. Close the lid and preheat for 15 minutes.
4. Place the marinated pork loin on the grill grate and cook until the temperature registers to 145°F. Cook for 2 to 3 hours on low heat.
5. Meanwhile, place the marinade in a saucepan. Place the saucepan in the grill and allow to simmer until the sauce has reduced.
6. Before taking the meat out, baste the pork with the reduced marinade.
7. Allow to rest for 10 minutes before slicing.

NUTRITION INFORMATION:

Calories per serving: 203 ; Protein: 26.4g; Carbs: 15.4g; Fat: 3.6g Sugar: 14.6g

Competition Style BBQ Pork Ribs

Serves: 6   **Cooking Time:** 2 hours

INGREDIENTS:

- 2 racks of St. Louis-style ribs
- 1 cup Traeger Pork and Poultry Rub
- 1/8 cup brown sugar
- 4 tablespoons butter
- 4 tablespoons agave
- 1 bottle Traeger Sweet and Heat BBQ Sauce

DIRECTIONS:

1. Place the ribs in working surface and remove the thin film of connective tissues covering it. In a smaller bowl, combine the Traeger Pork and Poultry Rub, brown sugar, butter, and agave. Mix until well combined.
2. Massage the rub onto the ribs and allow to rest in the fridge for at least 2 hours.
3. When ready to cook, fire the Traeger Grill to 225°F. Use desired wood pellets when cooking the ribs. Close the lid and preheat for 15 minutes.
4. Place the ribs on the grill grate and close the lid. Smoke for 1 hour and 30 minutes. Make sure to flip the ribs halfway through the cooking time.
5. Ten minutes before the cooking time ends, brush the ribs with BBQ sauce.
6. Remove from the grill and allow to rest before slicing.

NUTRITION INFORMATION:

Calories per serving: 399 ; Protein: 47.2g; Carbs: 3.5g; Fat: 20.5g Sugar: 2.3g

Smoked Apple BBQ Ribs

☕ **Serves:** 6   ⊕ **Cooking Time:** 2 hours

INGREDIENTS:

- 2 racks St. Louis-style ribs
- ¼ cup Traeger Big Game Rub
- 1 cup apple juice
- A bottle of Traeger BBQ Sauce

DIRECTIONS:

1. Place the ribs on a working surface and remove the film of connective tissues covering it.
2. In another bowl, mix the Game Rub and apple juice until well-combined.
3. Massage the rub on to the ribs and allow to rest in the fridge for at least 2 hours.
4. When ready to cook, fire the Traeger Grill to 225°F. Use apple wood pellets when cooking the ribs. Close the lid and preheat for 15 minutes.
5. Place the ribs on the grill grate and close the lid. Smoke for 1 hour and 30 minutes. Make sure to flip the ribs halfway through the cooking time.
6. Ten minutes before the cooking time ends, brush the ribs with BBQ sauce.
7. Remove from the grill and allow to rest before slicing.

NUTRITION INFORMATION:

Calories per serving: 337 ; Protein: 47.1g; Carbs: 4.7 g; Fat: 12.9g Sugar: 4g

Citrus-Brined Pork Roast

Serves: 6   **Cooking Time:** 45 minutes

INGREDIENTS:

- ½ cup salt
- ¼ cup brown sugar
- 3 cloves of garlic, minced
- 2 dried bay leaves
- 6 peppercorns
- 1 lemon, juiced
- ½ teaspoon dried fennel seeds
- ½ teaspoon red pepper flakes
- ½ cup apple juice
- ½ cup orange juice
- 5 pounds pork loin
- 2 tablespoons extra virgin olive oil

DIRECTIONS:

1. In a bowl, combine the salt, brown sugar, garlic, bay leaves, peppercorns, lemon juice, fennel seeds, pepper flakes, apple juice, and orange juice. Mix to form a paste rub.
2. Rub the mixture on to the pork loin and allow to marinate for at least 2 hours in the fridge. Add in the oil.
3. When ready to cook, fire the Traeger Grill to 300°F. Use apple wood pellets when cooking. Close the lid and preheat for 15 minutes.
4. Place the seasoned pork loin on the grill grate and close the lid. Cook for 45 minutes. Make sure to flip the pork halfway through the cooking time.

NUTRITION INFORMATION:

Calories per serving: 869; Protein: 97.2g; Carbs: 15.2g; Fat: 43.9g Sugar: 13g

Pineapple Pork BBQ

Serves: 4   **Cooking Time:** 60 minutes

INGREDIENTS:

- 1-pound pork sirloin
- 4 cups pineapple juice
- 3 cloves garlic, minced
- 1 cup carne asada marinade
- 2 tablespoons salt
- 1 teaspoon ground black pepper

DIRECTIONS:

1. Place all ingredients in a bowl. Massage the pork sirloin to coat with all ingredients. Place inside the fridge to marinate for at least 2 hours.
2. When ready to cook, fire the Traeger Grill to 300°F. Use desired wood pellets when cooking the ribs. Close the lid and preheat for 15 minutes.
3. Place the pork sirloin on the grill grate and cook for 45 to 60 minutes. Make sure to flip the pork halfway through the cooking time.
4. At the same time when you put the pork on the grill grate, place the marinade in a pan and place inside the smoker. Allow the marinade to cook and reduce.
5. Baste the pork sirloin with the reduced marinade before the cooking time ends.
6. Allow to rest before slicing.

NUTRITION INFORMATION:

Calories per serving: 347; Protein: 33.4 g; Carbs: 45.8 g; Fat: 4.2g Sugar: 36g

BBQ Spareribs with Mandarin Glaze

Serves: 6   **Cooking Time:** 60 minutes

INGREDIENTS:

- 3 large spareribs, membrane removed
- 3 tablespoons yellow mustard
- 1 tablespoons Worcestershire sauce
- 1 cup honey
- 1 ½ cup brown sugar
- 13 ounces Traeger Mandarin Glaze
- 1 teaspoon sesame oil
- 1 teaspoon soy sauce
- 1 teaspoon garlic powder

DIRECTIONS:

1. Place the spareribs on a working surface and carefully remove the connective tissue membrane that covers the ribs.
2. In another bowl, mix together the rest of the ingredients until well combined. Massage the spice mixture on to the spareribs. Allow to rest in the fridge for at least 3 hours.
3. When ready to cook, fire the Traeger Grill to 300ºF. Use hickory wood pellets when cooking the ribs. Close the lid and preheat for 15 minutes.
4. Place the seasoned ribs on the grill grate and cover the lid. Cook for 60 minutes.
5. Once cooked, allow to rest before slicing.

NUTRITION INFORMATION:

Calories per serving: 1263 ; Protein: 36.9g; Carbs: 110.3g; Fat: 76.8g Sugar: 107g

Smoked Pork Sausages

Serves: 6   **Cooking Time:** 1 hour

INGREDIENTS:

- 3 pounds ground pork
- ½ tablespoon ground mustard
- 1 tablespoon onion powder
- 1 tablespoon garlic powder
- 1 teaspoon pink curing salt
- 1 teaspoon salt
- 1 teaspoon black pepper
- ¼ cup ice water
- Hog casings, soaked and rinsed in cold water

DIRECTIONS:

1. Mix all ingredients except for the hog casings in a bowl. Using your hands, mix until all ingredients are well-combined.
2. Using a sausage stuffer, stuff the hog casings with the pork mixture.
3. Measure 4 inches of the stuffed hog casing and twist to form into a sausage. Repeat the process until you create sausage links.
4. When ready to cook, fire the Traeger Grill to 225°F. Use apple wood pellets when cooking the ribs. Close the lid and preheat for 15 minutes.
5. Place the sausage links on the grill grate and cook for 1 hour or until the internal temperature of the sausage reads at 155°F.
6. Allow to rest before slicing.

NUTRITION INFORMATION:

Calories per serving: 688; Protein: 58.9g; Carbs: 2.7g; Fat: 47.3g Sugar: 0.2g

Braised Pork Chile Verde

☕ **Serves:** 6   🕐 **Cooking Time:** 40 minutes

INGREDIENTS:

- 3 pounds pork shoulder, bone removed and cut into ½ inch cubes
- 1 tablespoon all-purpose flour   • Salt and pepper to taste
- 1-pound tomatillos, husked and washed
- 2 jalapenos, chopped
- 1 medium yellow onion, peeled and cut into chunks
- 4 cloves of garlic   • 1 tablespoon cumin
- 4 tablespoons extra virgin olive oil   • 1 tablespoon oregano
- 2 cup chicken stock   • ½ lime, juiced
- 2 cans green chilies   • ¼ cup cilantro

DIRECTIONS:

1. Place the pork shoulder chunks in a bowl and toss with flour. Season with salt and pepper to taste.
2. When ready to cook, fire the Traeger Grill to 500ºF. Use desired wood pellets when cooking. Place a large cast iron skillet on the bottom rack of the grill. Close the lid and preheat for 15 minutes.
3. Place the tomatillos, jalapeno, onion, and garlic on a sheet tray lined with foil and drizzle with 2 tablespoon olive oil. Season with salt and pepper to taste.
4. Place the remaining olive oil in the heated cast iron skillet and cook the pork shoulder. Spread the meat evenly then close.
5. Before closing the lid, place the vegetables in the tray on the grill rack. Close the lid of the grill.
6. Cook for 20 minutes without opening the lid or stirring the pork. After 20 minutes, remove the vegetables from the grill and transfer to a blender. Pulse until smooth and pour into the pan with the pork.
7. Stir in the chicken stock, green chilies, cumin, oregano, and lime juice. Season with salt and pepper to taste.
8. Close the grill lid and cook for another 20 minutes.
9. Once cooked, stir in the cilantro.

NUTRITION INFORMATION:

Calories per serving: 389; Protein: 28.5g; Carbs: 4.5g; Fat: 24.3g Sugar: 2.1g

Apricot Pork Tenderloin

☕ **Serves:** 4   🕐 **Cooking Time:** 1 ½ hours

INGREDIENTS:

- 2 pounds pork tenderloin
- 3 ounces Traeger Big Game Rub
- 1 cup Traeger Apricot BBQ Sauce

DIRECTIONS:

1. Place the pork tenderloin in a bowl and massage with the Big Game Rub. Allow to rest in the fridge for 2 hours.
2. When ready to cook, fire the Traeger Grill to 355ºF. Use desired wood pellets when cooking. Close the lid and preheat for 15 minutes.
3. Place the seasoned pork tenderloin on the grill grate and close the lid. Cook for 1 ½ hours. Make sure to flip the pork tenderloin halfway through the cooking time.
4. 10 minutes before the cooking time ends, baste the meat with the apricot BBQ sauce.
5. Allow to rest for 10 minutes before slicing.

NUTRITION INFORMATION:

Calories per serving: 426; Protein: 65.3g; Carbs: 20.4g; Fat: 8.4g Sugar: 17.8g

BBQ Brown Sugar Bacon

Serves: 3   **Cooking Time:** 30 minutes

INGREDIENTS:

- ½ cup brown sugar
- 1 tablespoon fennel, ground
- 2 teaspoons salt
- 1 teaspoon black pepper
- 1-pound pork belly, sliced thinly into bacon

DIRECTIONS:

1. Place all ingredients in a bowl and mix until well combined. Allow seasoned pork to rest in the fridge for at least 3 hours.
2. When ready to cook, fire the Traeger Grill to 255ºF. Use maple wood pellets when cooking. Close the lid and preheat for 15 minutes.
3. Place the bacon on the grill grate and close the lid. Smoke for 20 to 30 minutes.

NUTRITION INFORMATION:

Calories per serving: 331 ; Protein: 26.2g; Carbs: 39.7g; Fat: 8.5g Sugar: 26.7g

Smoked Pulled Pork

Serves: 4   **Cooking Time:** 6 hours

INGREDIENTS:

- 2 pounds bone-in pork shoulder
- Traeger Big Game Rub
- 2 cups apple cider
- Traeger 'Que BBQ Sauce

DIRECTIONS:

1. Place the pork shoulder in a bowl and remove excess fat and season with the Big Game Rub.
2. When ready to cook, fire the Traeger Grill to 250°F. Use maple wood pellets when cooking. Close the lid and preheat for 15 minutes.
3. Place pork on the grill grate for 5 hours or until the internal temperature reaches 160°F.
4. Remove the pork from the grill and allow to rest.
5. On a baking sheet, stack 4 pieces of aluminum foil on top of each other. Place the pork in the center of the foil and bring up the sides of the foil to create a sleeve around the pork. Scrimp the edges to ensure that any liquid does not escape from the sleeve. Pour over the apple cider.
6. Place the foil-wrapped pork on the grill and cook for another 3 hours at 204°F.
7. Remove from the grill and allow to rest.
8. Remove the pork from the foil sleeve and transfer to a plate, use forks to shred the meat. Discard the bones if any.
9. Once the pork has been shredded pour over the BBQ sauce.

NUTRITION INFORMATION:

Calories per serving: 634; Protein: 57g; Carbs: 7.6g; Fat: 40.2g Sugar: 5.7g

Fall-Of-The-Bone BBQ Ribs

🍵 **Serves:** 10   🕐 **Cooking Time:** 1 ½ hours

INGREDIENTS:

- 2/3 cup brown sugar
- ½ cup paprika
- 1/3 cup garlic powder
- 2 tablespoons onion powder
- 2 tablespoons chili powder
- 1 tablespoon cayenne pepper
- 1 tablespoon ground black pepper
- 1 teaspoon dried oregano
- 1 teaspoon ground cumin
- 1 ½ cup apple juice
- 4 rack baby back ribs
- ½ cup grape juice
- ½ cup honey
- 2 tablespoons soy sauce

DIRECTIONS:

1. Place all ingredients in a bowl except for the grape juice, honey, and soy sauce. Massage the meat with the marinade. Allow to rest in the fridge for at least 4 hours.
2. When ready to cook, fire the Traeger Grill to 275ºF. Use maple wood pellets when cooking. Close the lid and preheat for 15 minutes.
3. Place the seasoned grill on the grill grate and cook for 1 hour and 30 minutes.
4. Meanwhile, mix together the grape juice, honey, and soy sauce.
5. Once the ribs are cooked, remove from the grill, and allow to rest before slicing.
6. Pour over the sauce before serving.

NUTRITION INFORMATION:

Calories per serving: 923; Protein: 57.1g; Carbs: 47.7g; Fat:25 g Sugar: 23.1g

Cocoa-Crusted Pork Tenderloin

☕ **Serves:** 1   🕐 **Cooking Time:** 50 minutes

INGREDIENTS:

- 1 pork tenderloin
- ½ teaspoon fennel, ground
- 2 teaspoons cocoa powder, unsweetened
- 1 teaspoon smoked paprika
- ½ teaspoon salt
- ½ teaspoon black pepper
- 1 tablespoon extra-virgin olive oil

DIRECTIONS:

1. Place the pork tenderloin on a working surface and remove the membrane from the loin.
2. Mix the remaining ingredients in a small bowl to create the spice rub. Massage the pork tenderloin with the spice mixture and allow to rest in the fridge for at least 30 minutes.
3. When ready to cook, fire the Traeger Grill to 500°F. Use maple wood pellets when cooking. Close the lid and preheat for 15 minutes.
4. Place the loin on the grill grate and cook for 50 minutes or until the internal temperature reads at 145°F.
5. Remove from the grill and allow to rest for 10 minutes before slicing.

NUTRITION INFORMATION:

Calories per serving: 552; Protein: 88.5g; Carbs: 4.8g; Fat: 18.5g Sugar: 0.4g

Apple Bourbon Glazed Ham

Serves: 6   **Cooking Time:** 60 minutes

INGREDIENTS:

- 1 cup apple jelly
- 2 tablespoons Dijon mustard
- 2 tablespoons bourbon
- 2 tablespoons lemon juice
- ½ teaspoon ground cloves
- 2 cups apple juice
- 1 large ham

DIRECTIONS:

1. Fire the Traeger Grill to 500°F. Use maple wood pellets when cooking. Close the lid and preheat for 15 minutes.
2. In a small saucepan, combine the apple jelly, mustard, bourbon, lemon juice, cloves, and apple juice. Cook on low heat to melt the apple jelly. Cook for 5 minutes and set aside.
3. Place the ham in a baking tray and glaze with the reserved mixture.
4. Place on the grill rack and cook for 60 minutes.
5. Once the ham is cooked, remove from the grill, and allow to rest for 20 minutes before slicing.
6. Pour over the remaining glaze.

NUTRITION INFORMATION:

Calories per serving: 283; Protein: 38.7 g; Carbs: 14.7g; Fat: 8g Sugar: 10g

BEEF, LAMB, AND GOAT RECIPES

Pastrami Short Ribs

☕ **Serves:** 4   🕐 **Cooking Time:** 3 ½ hours

INGREDIENTS:

- 2 quarts water
- 1/3 cup salt
- 2 teaspoon pink salt
- ¼ cup brown sugar
- 4 garlic
- 4 tablespoons coriander seeds
- 3 tablespoons peppercorns
- 2 teaspoons mustard seeds
- 2 tablespoons extra virgin olive oil
- 1 large ginger ale
- 2 pounds beef short ribs

DIRECTIONS:

1. Place all ingredients except for the oil, ginger ale, and short ribs in a large bowl. Mix until well-combined. Add in the short ribs. Marinate the short ribs in the fridge for at least 12 hours.
2. When ready to cook, fire the Traeger Grill to 300°F. Use desired wood pellets when cooking. Close the lid and preheat for 15 minutes.
3. Place the short ribs on the grill grate and smoke for 2 hours. Drizzle with oil.
4. Transfer the ribs on a roasting pan and pour enough ginger ale all over the ribs. Cover the pan with foil.
5. Place in the grill and increase the temperature to 350°F and cook for 1 ½ hours.

NUTRITION INFORMATION:

Calories per serving: 521 ; Protein: 46.7g; Carbs: 16.9g; Fat: 30.1g Sugar: 13.7g

Grilled Butter Basted Porterhouse Steak

☕ **Serves:**4   ⊕ **Cooking Time:** 8 minutes

INGREDIENTS:

- 4 tablespoons melted butter
- 2 tablespoons Worcestershire sauce
- 2 tablespoons Dijon mustard
- Traeger Prime Rib Rub, as needed
- 2 porterhouse steaks, 1 ½ inch thick

DIRECTIONS:

1. Fire the Traeger Grill to 255ºF. Use desired wood pellets when cooking. Close the lid and preheat for 15 minutes.
2. In a bowl, mix the butter, Worcestershire sauce, mustard, and Prime Rib Rub.
3. Massage all over the steak on all sides. Allow steak to rest for an hour before cooking.
4. When ready to cook, fire the Traeger Grill to 500ºF. Use desired wood pellets when cooking. Close the lid and preheat for 15 minutes.
5. Place the steaks on the grill grates and cook for 4 minutes on each side or until the internal temperature reads at 130ºF for medium rare steaks.
6. Remove from the grill and allow to rest for 10 minutes before slicing.

NUTRITION INFORMATION:

Calories per serving: 515 ; Protein: 65.3g; Carbs: 2.1g; Fat: 27.7g Sugar: 0.9g

Braised Mediterranean Beef Brisket

☕ **Serves:** 16   ⊕ **Cooking Time:** 5 hours

INGREDIENTS:

- 3 tablespoons dried rosemary
- 2 tablespoons cumin seeds, ground
- 2 tablespoons dried coriander
- 1 tablespoon dried oregano
- 2 teaspoons ground cinnamon
- ½ teaspoon salt
- 8 pounds beef brisket, sliced into chunks
- 1 cup beef stock

DIRECTIONS:

1. Mix the rosemary, cumin, coriander, oregano, cinnamon, and salt in a bowl.
2. Massage the spice mix into the beef brisket and allow to rest in the fridge for 12 hours.
3. When ready to cook, fire the Traeger Grill to 180°F. Use desired wood pellets when cooking. Close the lid and preheat for 15 minutes.
4. Place the brisket fat side down on the grill grate and cook for 4 hours.
5. After 4 hours, turn up the heat to 250°F.
6. Continue cooking the beef brisket until the internal temperature reaches 160°F. Remove and place on a foil. Crimp the edges of the foil to create a sleeve. Pour in the beef stock.
7. Return the brisket in the foil sleeve and continue cooking for another hour.

NUTRITION INFORMATION:

Calories per serving: 453 ; Protein: 33.5g; Carbs: 1g; Fat: 34g Sugar: 0.1g

Brined Smoked Brisket

Serves: 6   **Cooking Time:** 6 hours and 30 minutes

INGREDIENTS:

- 1 cup brown sugar
- ½ cup salt
- 1 flat cut brisket
- ¼ cup Traeger Beef Rub

DIRECTIONS:

1. Make the brine by dissolving the sugar and salt in 6 quarts hot water. Allow to cool at room temperature and place the brisket in the solution. Place in the fridge and allow to marinate for 12 hours.
2. Remove the brisket from the brine and pat dry with paper towel. Sprinkle with the Traeger Beef Rub and massage until all surfaces are coated.
3. When ready to cook, fire the Traeger Grill to 250ºF. Use desired wood pellets when cooking. Close the lid and preheat for 15 minutes.
4. Place the brisket on the grill grate and cook for 4 hours. After 3 hours, double wrap the brisket in foil and turn the temperature to 275ºF and cook for another 3 hours.
5. Unwrap the brisket and grill for 30 minutes more.
6. Remove the brisket from the grill and allow to rest before slicing.

NUTRITION INFORMATION:

Calories per serving: 364; Protein: 48.7 g; Carbs: 16.6g; Fat: 11.6g Sugar: 12.3g

BBQ Brisket with Coffee Rub

Serves: 10   **Cooking Time:** 6 hours

INGREDIENTS:

- 5 pounds whole packer brisket
- 2 tablespoons Traeger Coffee Rub
- 1 cup water
- 2 tablespoons salt

DIRECTIONS:

1. Trim the brisket and remove any membrane. Leave a ¼" inch cap on the bottom.
2. In a bowl, combine the coffee rub, water, and salt until dissolved.
3. Season the brisket with the spice rub and allow to rest in the fridge for 3 hours.
4. When ready to cook, fire the Traeger Grill to 250°F. Use desired wood pellets when cooking. Close the lid and preheat for 15 minutes.
5. Place the brisket on the grill grate and close the lid. Cook for 6 hours or until the internal temperature reaches 160°F.
6. Wrap the brisket in aluminum foil and increase the temperature to 275°F. Cook for another 3 hours.

NUTRITION INFORMATION:

Calories per serving: 352; Protein: 47g; Carbs: 0g; Fat: 16.7g Sugar: 0g

Smoked Texas BBQ Brisket

Serves: 4   **Cooking Time:** 5 hours

INGREDIENTS:

- 6 pounds whole packer brisket
- Commercial BBQ rub of your choice

DIRECTIONS:

1. Trim the brisket from any membrane and loose fat. Trim the fat side to ¼ inch thick.
2. Season all sides of the brisket with the BBQ rub and allow to rest for 30 minutes inside the fridge.
3. When ready to cook, fire the Traeger Grill to 275°F. Use mesquite wood pellets when cooking. Close the lid and preheat for 15 minutes.
4. Place the brisket fat side up on the grill grate and cook for 5 hours or until the internal temperature reaches 165°F.
5. Once cooked, remove the brisket from the grill and allow to rest before slicing.

NUTRITION INFORMATION:

Calories per serving: 703; Protein: 93.9g; Carbs: 0 g; Fat: 33.4g Sugar: 0g

Roasted Leg of Lamb

🍵 **Serves:** 9   ⊕ **Cooking Time:** 2 hours

INGREDIENTS:

- 2 teaspoons extra virgin olive oil
- 1 tablespoon crushed garlic
- 7 pounds bone-in leg of lamb
- 4 cloves of garlic, sliced lengthwise
- 4 sprig rosemary, cut into 1-inch pieces
- 2 lemons, sliced
- Salt and pepper to taste

DIRECTIONS:

1. Combine olive oil and crushed garlic. Rub the mixture on the leg of lamb.
2. Make small perforations in the lamb using a sharp knife and stuff the slivered garlic and rosemary sprigs.
3. Zest and juice the lemons and sprinkle over the lamb. Season with salt and pepper to taste.
4. When ready to cook, fire the Traeger Grill to 500ºF. Use desired wood pellets when cooking. Close the lid and preheat for 15 minutes.
5. Place the seasoned leg of lamb on the grill grate and reduce the grill to 350ºF. Cook for 2 hours.
6. Let the lamb rest for 15 minutes before carving.

NUTRITION INFORMATION:
Calories per serving: 439; Protein: 74.1g; Carbs: 2g; Fat: 14.9g Sugar: 0.6g

Grilled Lamb Kabobs

Serves: 7   **Cooking Time:** 16 minutes

INGREDIENTS:

- ½ cup olive oil
- ½ tablespoon salt
- 2 teaspoons black pepper
- 2 tablespoons chopped mint
- ½ tablespoon cilantro, chopped
- 1 teaspoon cumin
- ½ cup lemon juice
- 3 pounds boneless leg of lamb, cut into 2-inch cubes
- 15 apricots, halved and seeded
- 5 onions, cut into wedges

DIRECTIONS:

1. In a bowl, combine the oil, salt, pepper, mint, cilantro, cumin, and lemon juice.
2. Massage the mixture on to the lamb shoulder and allow to marinate in the fridge for at least 2 hours.
3. Remove the lamb from the marinade and thread the lamb, apricots, and red onion alternatingly on a skewer.
4. When ready to cook, fire the Traeger Grill to 400ºF. Use desired wood pellets when cooking. Close the lid and preheat for 15 minutes.
5. Place the skewers on the grill grate and cook for 8 minutes on each side.
6. Remove from the grill.

NUTRITION INFORMATION:

Calories per serving: 652; Protein: 53.9g; Carbs: 38.1g; Fat: 31.8g Sugar: 29.4g

Braised Lamb Shank

Serves: 6   **Cooking Time:** 4 hours

INGREDIENTS:

- 6 whole lamb shanks
- Traeger Prime Rib Rub
- 1 cup beef broth
- 1 cup red wine
- 4 sprig rosemary and thyme

DIRECTIONS:

1. Season the lamb shanks with Traeger Prime Rib Rub.
2. When ready to cook, fire the Traeger Grill to 500°F. Use desired wood pellets when cooking. Close the lid and preheat for 15 minutes.
3. Place the lamb shanks directly on the grill grate and cook for 20 minutes or until the surface browns.
4. Transfer the shanks to a Dutch oven and pour in beef broth.
5. Place the Dutch oven back on the grill grate and reduce the temperature to 325°F. Cook for another 3 to 4 hours.

NUTRITION INFORMATION:

Calories per serving: 532 ; Protein: 55.2g; Carbs: 10.2g; Fat: 21.4g Sugar: 2.3g

Smoked Lamb Leg with Salsa Verde

Serves: 6   **Cooking Time:** 3 hours

INGREDIENTS:

- 2 tablespoons oil
- 1 whole leg of lamb, fat trimmed and cut into chunks
- Salt to taste
- 6 cloves green garlic, unpeeled
- 1-pound tomatillos, husked and washed
- 1 small yellow onion, quartered
- 5 whole serrano chili peppers
- 1 tablespoon capers, drained
- ¼ cup cilantro, finely chopped
- ½ teaspoon sugar
- 1 cup chicken broth
- 3 tablespoons lime juice, freshly squeezed

DIRECTIONS:

1. Fire the Traeger Grill to 500ºF. Use desired wood pellets when cooking. Close the lid and preheat for 15 minutes. Place a Dutch oven on the grill grate and add oil.
2. Put the lamb in the Dutch oven and season with salt to taste. Stir once then close the lid.
3. Place the garlic, tomatillos, onion, serrano peppers, and capers in a parchment-lined baking tray. Season with salt to taste and drizzle with olive oil.
4. Place in the grill and cook for 15 minutes.
5. Remove the vegetables from the grill and transfer to a blender. Add cilantro and sugar. Season with more salt if needed. Pulse until smooth then set aside.
6. Pour the mixture into the Dutch oven and add in chicken broth and lime juice.
7. Allow to cook for 3 hours.

NUTRITION INFORMATION:

Calories per serving: 430; Protein: 56.4g; Carbs: 7.8g; Fat: 18.4g Sugar: 3.9g

Grilled Lamb Chops with Rosemary

🍵 **Serves:** 4   ⊕ **Cooking Time:** 12 minutes

INGREDIENTS:

- ½ cup extra virgin olive oil
- ¼ cup coarsely chopped onion
- 2 cloves of garlic, minced
- 2 tablespoons soy sauce
- 2 tablespoons balsamic vinegar
- 1 tablespoon fresh rosemary
- 2 teaspoons Dijon mustard
- 1 teaspoon Worcestershire sauce
- Salt and pepper to taste
- 4 lamb chops (8 ounce each)

DIRECTIONS:

1. Heat oil in a saucepan over medium flame and sauté the onion and garlic until fragrant. Place in food processor together with the soy sauce, vinegar, rosemary, mustard, Worcestershire sauce, salt, and pepper. Pulse until smooth. Set aside.
2. Fire the Traeger Grill to 500°F. Use desired wood pellets when cooking. Close the lid and preheat for 15 minutes.
3. Brush the lamb chops on both sides with the paste.
4. Place on the grill grates and cook for 6 minutes per side or until the internal temperature reaches 135°F for medium rare.
5. Serve with the paste if you have leftover.

NUTRITION INFORMATION: Calories per serving: 442; Protein: 16.7g; Carbs: 6.1g; Fat:38.5 g Sugar: 3.7g

Bison Tomahawk Steak

Serves: 4   **Cooking Time:** 12 minutes

INGREDIENTS:

- 2 ½ whole bone-in buffalo rib-eye steak
- 2 teaspoons cherrywood smoked salt
- 1 ½ tablespoons black pepper

DIRECTIONS:

1. Fire the Traeger Grill to 450°F. Use desired wood pellets when cooking. Close the lid and preheat for 15 minutes.
2. Season the rib-eye steak with salt and pepper to taste.
3. Place the steak directly on the grill grate. Grill for 6 minutes on each side or until the internal temperature reaches 140°F.
4. Remove from the grill and allow to rest before slicing.

NUTRITION INFORMATION:

Calories per serving: 751; Protein: 51.6g; Carbs: 1.7g; Fat: 60.1g; Sugar: 0.02g

Braised Elk Shank

Serves: 6   **Cooking Time:** 4 hours and 10 minutes

INGREDIENTS:

- 3 elk shanks
- Salt and pepper to taste
- 3 tablespoons canola oil
- 2 whole onions, halved
- 4 cloves of garlic, minced
- 2 dried bay leaves
- 2 cups red wine
- 1 sprig of rosemary
- 2 carrots, peeled and halved lengthwise
- 1 bunch fresh thyme
- 3 quarts beef stock

DIRECTIONS:

1. Fire the Traeger Grill to 500ºF. Use desired wood pellets when cooking. Place a cast-iron pan on the grill grate. Close the lid and preheat for 15 minutes.
2. Season the shanks with salt and pepper. Place canola oil in the heated cast iron and place the shanks. Close the grill lid and cook for five minutes on each side.
3. Add the onions and garlic and sauté for 1 minute.
4. Stir in the rest of the ingredients.
5. Close the grill lid and cook for 4 hours until soft.

NUTRITION INFORMATION:

Calories per serving: 331 ; Protein: 47.2g; Carbs: 11.5g; Fat: 11.2g Sugar: 5.4g

Baked Venison Meatloaf

☕ **Serves:** 6   ⊕ **Cooking Time:** 1 hour and 30 minutes

INGREDIENTS:

- 2 pounds venison, ground
- 1-pound pork, ground
- 1 cup breadcrumbs
- 1 cup milk
- 2 tablespoons onion, diced
- 3 tablespoons salt
- 1 tablespoon black pepper
- ½ tablespoon thyme
- 1 ½ pounds parsnips, chopped
- 1 ½ pounds russet potatoes, chopped
- ¼ cup butter

DIRECTIONS:

1. Fire the Traeger Grill to 500ºF. Use desired wood pellets when cooking. Close the lid and preheat for 15 minutes.
2. Combine all ingredients in a bowl. Place the mixture in a greased loaf pan.
3. Place in the Traeger Grill and cook for 1 hour and 30 minutes or until the internal temperature reads at 160ºF.

NUTRITION INFORMATION:

Calories per serving: 668 ; Protein: 70.4g; Carbs: 45.7 g; Fat: 22g Sugar: 8.7g

Roasted Venison Tenderloin

☕ **Serves:** 4   ⊕ **Cooking Time:** 20 minutes

INGREDIENTS:

- 2 pounds venison
- ¼ cup dry red wine
- 2 cloves garlic, minced
- 2 tablespoons soy sauce
- 1 ½ tablespoons red wine vinegar
- 1 tablespoon rosemary
- 1 teaspoon black pepper
- ½ cup olive oil
- Salt to taste

DIRECTIONS:

1. Remove the membrane covering the venison. Set aside.
2. Mix the rest of the ingredients in a bowl. Place the venison in the bowl and allow to marinate for at least 5 hours in the fridge.
3. Fire the Traeger Grill to 500°F. Use desired wood pellets when cooking. Close the lid and preheat for 15 minutes.
4. Remove the venison from the marinade and pat dry using a paper towel.
5. Place on the grill grate and cook for 10 minutes on each side for medium rare.

NUTRITION INFORMATION:

Calories per serving: 611 ; Protein: 68.4g; Carbs: 3.1g; Fat: 34.4g Sugar: 1.6g

Grilled Venison Kabob

Serves: 6   **Cooking Time:** 15 minutes

INGREDIENTS:

- 1 venison, black strap steaks cut into large cubes
- 2 whole red onion, quartered
- 2 whole green bell pepper, sliced into big squares
- Oil as needs
- Salt and pepper to taste

DIRECTIONS:

1. Place all ingredients in a mixing bowl. Toss to coat the meat and vegetables with the oil and seasoning.
2. Thread the meat and vegetables into metal skewers in an alternating manner.
3. Fire the Traeger Grill to 500°F. Use desired wood pellets when cooking. Close the lid and preheat for 15 minutes.
4. Place the kabobs on the grill grate and cook for 15 minutes. Make sure to turn once halfway through the cooking time.
5. Remove from the grill and serve with yogurt if desired.

NUTRITION INFORMATION:

Calories per serving: 267; Protein: 32.4g; Carbs: 10.1g; Fat: 10.4g Sugar:4.8 g

Sweetheart Steak

☕ **Serves:** 1   ⊕ **Cooking Time:** 14 minutes

INGREDIENTS:

- 20 ounces boneless strip steak, butterflied
- 2 ounces pure sea salt
- 2 teaspoons black pepper
- 2 tablespoons raw dark chocolate, finely chopped
- ½ tablespoon extra-virgin olive oil

DIRECTIONS:

1. On a cutting board, trim the meat into heart shape using a sharp knife. Set aside.
2. In a smaller bowl, combine the rest of the ingredients to create a spice rub mix.
3. Rub onto the steak and massage until well-seasoned.
4. When ready to cook, fire the Traeger Grill to 450°F. Use desired wood pellets when cooking. Close the lid and preheat for 15 minutes.
5. Grill the steak for 7 minutes on each side.
6. Allow to rest for 5 minutes before slicing.

NUTRITION INFORMATION:

Calories per serving: 727 ; Protein: 132.7g; Carbs: 8.8 g; Fat: 18.5g Sugar: 5.2g

Bloody Mary Flank Steak

Serves: 3   **Cooking Time:** 14 minutes

INGREDIENTS:

- 2 cups Traeger Smoked Bloody Mary Mix or V8 Juice
- ½ cup vodka
- 1 whole lemon, juiced
- 3 cloves garlic, minced
- 1 tablespoon Worcestershire sauce
- 1 teaspoon ground black pepper
- 1 teaspoon celery salt
- ½ cup vegetable oil
- 1 ½ pound flank steak

DIRECTIONS:

1. Place all ingredients except for the flank steak in a bowl. Mix until well-combined.
2. Put the flank steak in a plastic bag and pour half of the marinade over. Marinate for at least 24 hours in the fridge.
3. When ready to cook, fire the Traeger Grill to 500ºF. Use desired wood pellets when cooking. Close the lid and preheat for 15 minutes.
4. Drain the flank steak and pat dry using a paper towel.
5. Place on the grill grate and cook for 7 minutes on each side.
6. Meanwhile, place the remaining marinade (unused) in a saucepan and heat until the sauce thickens.
7. Once the steak is cooked, remove from the grill, and allow to rest for 5 minutes before slicing.
8. Pour over the sauce.

NUTRITION INFORMATION:

Calories per serving: 719 ; Protein: 51.9g; Carbs: 15.4g; Fat: 51g Sugar: 6.9g

Rosemary Prime Rib

Serves: 8   **Cooking Time:** 1 hour

INGREDIENTS:

- 8 pounds whole ribeye roast
- 4 tablespoons olive oil
- 4 tablespoons peppercorns
- 3 whole rosemary sprigs
- ½ cup garlic, minced
- ½ cup smoked salt

DIRECTIONS:

1. Fire the Traeger Grill to 500°F. Use desired wood pellets when cooking. Close the lid and preheat for 15 minutes.
2. Cut the rib loin in half and sear the halves in oil over high heat until golden brown. Set aside.
3. Place the peppercorns in a bag and crush with a rolling pin. Next, strip the rosemary leaves from the stem and mix with garlic and salt.
4. Season the seared steak with the spice mixture.
5. Place in the grill and roast for 30 minutes and reduce the heat to 300°F. Cook for another 30 minutes.
6. Once cooked, remove from the grill, and allow to rest for 20 minutes before slicing.

NUTRITION INFORMATION:

Calories per serving: 954; Protein: 128.5g; Carbs: 4.1g; Fat: 47.7g Sugar: 0.3g

Traeger Tri-Tip Roast

Serves: 6   **Cooking Time:** 3 hours and 45 minutes

INGREDIENTS:

- 1 tri-tip roast
- Traeger 'Que BBQ Sauce, as needed
- Traeger Prime Rib Rub, as needed
- ½ cup beef broth

DIRECTIONS:

1. Marinate the tri-trip roast in the Traeger Que BBQ Sauce overnight inside the fridge.
2. Once ready to cook, remove the beef from the marinade and season with the Prime Rib Rub.
3. Fire the Traeger Grill to 180°F. Use desired wood pellets when cooking. Close the lid and preheat for 15 minutes.
4. Place the beef on the grill grate and cook for 3 hours.
5. Remove from the grill and place the beef on an aluminum foil sheet. Crimp the edges of the aluminum foil to create a sleeve.
6. Place the roast in the aluminum sleeve on the grill grate and pour over the beef broth.
7. Pour over the broth and increase the heat to 300°F. Cook for 45 minutes.

NUTRITION INFORMATION:

Calories per serving: 357; Protein: 48g; Carbs: 1.7g; Fat: 16g Sugar: 0g

VEGGIES RECIPES

Traeger Fries with Chipotle Ketchup

☕ **Serves:** 6   🕐 **Cooking Time:** 10 minutes

INGREDIENTS:

- 6 Yukon Gold potatoes, scrubbed and cut into thick strips
- 1 tablespoon Traeger Beef Rub
- 1 tablespoon extra-virgin olive oil
- 1 teaspoon onion powder
- 1 teaspoon garlic powder
- ½ cup chipotle peppers, chopped
- 1 cup ketchup
- 1 tablespoon sugar
- 1 tablespoon cumin
- 1 tablespoon chili powder
- 1 whole lime
- 2 tablespoons butter

DIRECTIONS:

1. Place the potatoes in a bowl and stir in the Traeger Beef Rub, olive oil, onion powder, and garlic powder. Toss to coat the potatoes with the spices.
2. Fire the Traeger Grill to 500°F. Use desired wood pellets when cooking. Close the lid and preheat for 15 minutes.
3. Place the potatoes on a baking sheet lined with foil.
4. Place on the grill grate and cook for 10 minutes.
5. Meanwhile, place the rest of the ingredients in a small bowl and mix until well-combined.
6. Serve the fries with the chipotle ketchup sauce.

NUTRITION INFORMATION:
Calories per serving: 387 ; Protein: 8.6g; Carbs: 79.3g; Fat: 5.6g Sugar: 13.7g

Roasted Peach Salsa

☕ **Serves:** 6   ⏲ **Cooking Time:** 10 minutes

INGREDIENTS:

- 6 whole peaches, pitted and halved
- 3 tomatoes, chopped
- 2 whole onions, chopped
- ½ cup cilantro, chopped
- 2 cloves garlic, minced
- 5 teaspoons apple cider vinegar
- ½ teaspoon salt
- ¼ teaspoon black pepper
- 2 tablespoons olive oil

DIRECTIONS:

1. Fire the Traeger Grill to 300ºF. Use desired wood pellets when cooking. Close the lid and preheat for 15 minutes.
2. Place the peaches on the grill grate and cook for 5 minutes on each side. Remove from the grill and allow to rest for 5 minutes.
3. Place the peaches, tomatoes, onion, and cilantro in a salad bowl. On a smaller bowl, stir in the garlic, apple cider vinegar, salt, pepper, and olive oil. Stir until well-combined. Pour into the salad and toss to coat.

NUTRITION INFORMATION:

Calories per serving: 155 ; Protein: 3.1g; Carbs: 27.6 g; Fat: 5.1g Sugar: 20g

Smoked Pumpkin Soup

Serves: 6   **Cooking Time:** 1 hour and 33 minutes

INGREDIENTS:

- 5 pounds pumpkin, seeded and sliced
- 3 tablespoons butter
- 1 onion, diced
- 2 cloves garlic, minced
- 1 tablespoon brown sugar
- 1 teaspoon paprika
- ¼ teaspoon ground cinnamon
- ¼ teaspoon ground nutmeg
- ½ cup apple cider
- 5 cups broth
- ½ cup cream

DIRECTIONS:

1. Fire the Traeger Grill to 180ºF. Use desired wood pellets when cooking. Close the lid and preheat for 15 minutes.
2. Place the pumpkin on the grill grate and smoke for an hour or until tender. Allow to cool.
3. Melt the butter in a large saucepan over medium heat and sauté the onion and garlic for 3 minutes. Stir in the rest of the ingredients including the smoked pumpkin. Cook for another 30 minutes.
4. Transfer to a blender and pulse until smooth.

NUTRITION INFORMATION:

Calories per serving: 246; Protein: 8.8g; Carbs: 32.2g; Fat: 11.4g Sugar: 15.5g

Roasted Green Beans with Bacon

Serves: 6   **Cooking Time:** 20 minutes

INGREDIENTS:

- 1-pound green beans
- 4 strips bacon, cut into small pieces
- 4 tablespoons extra virgin olive oil
- 2 cloves garlic, minced
- 1 teaspoon salt

DIRECTIONS:

1. Fire the Traeger Grill to 400°F. Use desired wood pellets when cooking. Close the lid and preheat for 15 minutes.
2. Toss all ingredients on a sheet tray and spread out evenly.
3. Place the tray on the grill grate and roast for 20 minutes.

NUTRITION INFORMATION:

Calories per serving: 65 ; Protein: 1.3g; Carbs: 3.8g; Fat: 5.3g Sugar: 0.6g

Grilled Baby Carrots and Fennel

Serves: 8   **Cooking Time:** 30 minutes

INGREDIENTS:

- 1-pound slender rainbow carrots, washed and peeled
- 2 whole fennel bulbs, chopped
- 2 tablespoons extra virgin olive oil
- 1 teaspoon salt
- Salt to taste

DIRECTIONS:

1. Fire the Traeger Grill to 500ºF. Use desired wood pellets when cooking. Close the lid and preheat for 15 minutes.
2. Place all ingredients in a sheet tray and toss to coat with oil and seasoning.
3. Place on the grill grate and cook for 30 minutes.

NUTRITION INFORMATION:

Calories per serving:52 ; Protein: 1.2g; Carbs: 8.9g; Fat: 1.7g Sugar: 4.3g

Roasted Hasselback Potatoes

Serves: 6   **Cooking Time:** 30 minutes

INGREDIENTS:

- 6 large russet potatoes
- 1-pound bacon
- ½ cup butter
- Salt to taste
- 1 cup cheddar cheese
- 3 whole scallions, chopped

DIRECTIONS:

1. Fire the Traeger Grill to 350ºF. Use desired wood pellets when cooking. Close the lid and preheat for 15 minutes.
2. Place two wooden spoons on either side of the potato and slice the potato into thin strips without completely cutting through the potato.
3. Chop the bacon into small pieces and place in between the cracks or slices of the potatoes.
4. Place potatoes in a cast iron skillet. Top the potatoes with butter, salt, and cheddar cheese.
5. Place the skillet on the grill grate and cook for 30 minutes. Make sure to baste the potatoes with melted cheese 10 minutes before the cooking time ends.

NUTRITION INFORMATION:

Calories per serving: 662; Protein: 16.1g; Carbs: 71.5g; Fat: 38g Sugar: 2.3g

Smoked Mashed Red Potatoes

Serves: 8   **Cooking Time:** 30 minutes

INGREDIENTS:

- 8 large potatoes
- Salt and pepper to taste
- ½ cup heavy cream
- ¼ cup butter

DIRECTIONS:

1. Fire the Traeger Grill to 180°F. Use desired wood pellets when cooking. Close the lid and preheat for 15 minutes.
2. Slice the potatoes into half and season with salt and pepper to taste. Place on a baking tray.
3. Place the tray with the potatoes on the grill grate and cook for 30 minutes. Be sure to flip the potatoes halfway through the cooking time.
4. Once cooked, remove from the grill and place on a bowl. Add the rest of the ingredients and mash until well-combined.

NUTRITION INFORMATION:

Calories per serving: 363 ; Protein: 7.8g; Carbs: 65.2g; Fat: 8.9g Sugar: 3.4g

Baked Sweet and Savory Yams

🍵 **Serves:** 6   🕐 **Cooking Time:** 55 minutes

INGREDIENTS:

- 3 pounds yams, scrubbed
- 3 tablespoons extra virgin olive oil
- Honey to taste
- Goat cheese as needed
- ½ cup brown sugar
- ½ cup pecans, chopped

DIRECTIONS:

1. Fire the Traeger Grill to 350°F. Use desired wood pellets when cooking. Close the lid and preheat for 15 minutes.
2. Poke holes on the yams using a fork. Wrap yams in foil and place on the grill grate. Cook for 45 minutes until tender.
3. Remove the yams from the grill and allow to cool. Once cooled, peel the yam and slice to ¼" rounds.
4. Place on a parchment-lined baking tray and brush with olive oil. Drizzle with honey, cheese, brown sugar, and pecans.
5. Place in the grill and cook for another 10 minutes.

NUTRITION INFORMATION:

Calories per serving: 421; Protein: 4.3g; Carbs: 82.4g; Fat: 9.3g Sugar:19.3 g

Grilled Romaine Caesar Salad

🍵 **Serves:** 6   ⊕ **Cooking Time:** 5 minutes

INGREDIENTS:

- ¼ cup extra virgin olive oil
- 2 cloves garlic, minced
- 1 teaspoon Dijon mustard
- 1 cup mayonnaise
- Salt and pepper to taste
- 2 head Romaine lettuce
- ¼ cup parmesan cheese
- Croutons, optional

DIRECTIONS:

1. In a small bowl, combine the olive oil, garlic, mustard, and mayonnaise. Season with salt and pepper to taste. Mix and set aside.
2. Cut the Romaine in half lengthwise leaving the ends intact so that it does not come apart.
3. Fire the Traeger Grill to 400°F. Use desired wood pellets when cooking. Close the lid and preheat for 15 minutes.
4. Brush the Romaine lettuce with oil and place cut side down on the grill grate. Cook for 5 minutes.
5. Once cooked, chop the lettuce and place on a bowl. Toss with the salad dressing, parmesan cheese, and croutons.

NUTRITION INFORMATION:
Calories per serving: 235 ; Protein: 7.5g; Carbs: 19.4 g; Fat: 9.7g Sugar: 8.3g

Salt-Crusted Baked Potatoes

Serves: 6   **Cooking Time:** 40 minutes

INGREDIENTS:

- 6 russet potatoes, scrubbed and dried
- 3 tablespoons oil
- 1 tablespoons salt
- Butter as needed
- Sour cream as needed

DIRECTIONS:

1. Fire the Traeger Grill to 400ºF. Use desired wood pellets when cooking. Close the lid and preheat for 15 minutes.
2. In a large bowl, coat the potatoes with oil and salt. Place seasoned potatoes on a baking tray.
3. Place the tray with potatoes on the grill grate.
4. Close the lid and grill for 40 minutes.
5. Serve with butter and sour cream.

NUTRITION INFORMATION:

Calories per serving: 363; Protein: 8g; Carbs: 66.8g; Fat: 8.6g Sugar: 2.3g

Roasted Butternut Squash

Serves: 4   **Cooking Time:** 30 minutes

INGREDIENTS:

- 2-pound butternut squash
- 3 tablespoon extra-virgin olive oil
- Traeger Veggie Rub, as needed

DIRECTIONS:

1. Fire the Traeger Grill to 350ºF. Use desired wood pellets when cooking. Close the lid and preheat for 15 minutes.
2. Slice the butternut squash into ½ inch thick and remove the seeds. Season with oil and veggie rub.
3. Place the seasoned squash in a baking tray.
4. Grill for 30 minutes.

NUTRITION INFORMATION:

Calories per serving: 131; Protein: 1.9g; Carbs: 23.6g; Fat: 4.7g Sugar: 0g

Roasted Sheet Pan Vegetables

☕ **Serves:** 6   ⊕ **Cooking Time:** 20 minutes

INGREDIENTS:

- 1 small purple cauliflower, cut into florets
- 1 small yellow cauliflower, cut into florets
- 4 cups butternut squash
- 2 cups mushroom, fresh
- 3 tablespoons extra virgin olive oil
- 2 teaspoons salt
- 2 teaspoons black pepper

DIRECTIONS:

1. Fire the Traeger Grill to 350°F. Use desired wood pellets when cooking. Close the lid and preheat for 15 minutes.
2. Place the vegetables in a baking tray and season with olive oil, salt, and pepper. Toss to coat all vegetables.
3. Place in the grill and cook for 20 minutes. Make sure to shake the tray halfway through the cooking time for even cooking.

NUTRITION INFORMATION:

Calories per serving: 101; Protein: 3.8g; Carbs: 16.9g; Fat: 3.5g Sugar: 4.4g

Smoked Hummus

Serves: 6   **Cooking Time:** 20 minutes

INGREDIENTS:

- 1 ½ cups chickpeas, rinsed and drained
- ¼ cup tahini
- 1 tablespoon garlic, minced
- 2 tablespoons extra virgin olive oil
- 1 teaspoon salt
- 4 tablespoons lemon juice

DIRECTIONS:

1. Fire the Traeger Grill to 350°F. Use desired wood pellets when cooking. Close the lid and preheat for 15 minutes.
2. Spread the chickpeas on a sheet tray and place on the grill grate. Smoke for 20 minutes.
3. Let the chickpeas cool at room temperature.
4. Place smoked chickpeas in a blender or food processor. Add in the rest of the ingredients. Pulse until smooth.
5. Serve with roasted vegetables if desired.

NUTRITION INFORMATION:

Calories per serving: 271; Protein: 12.1g; Carbs: 34.8g; Fat: 10.4g Sugar: 5.7g

Grilled Corn with Honey Butter

Serves: 6   **Cooking Time:** 10 minutes

INGREDIENTS:

- 6 pieces corn, husked
- 2 tablespoons olive oil
- Salt and pepper to taste
- ½ cup butter, room temperature
- ½ cup honey

DIRECTIONS:

1. Fire the Traeger Grill to 350°F. Use desired wood pellets when cooking. Close the lid and preheat for 15 minutes.
2. Brush the corn with oil and season with salt and pepper to taste.
3. Place the corn on the grill grate and cook for 10 minutes. Make sure to flip the corn halfway through the cooking time for even cooking.
4. Meanwhile, mix the butter and honey on a small bowl. Set aside.
5. Once the corn is cooked, remove from the grill and brush with the honey butter sauce.

NUTRITION INFORMATION:

Calories per serving: 387; Protein: 5g; Carbs: 51.2g; Fat: 21.6g Sugar: 28.2g

Baked Cheesy Corn Pudding

☕ **Serves:** 6   ⊕ **Cooking Time:** 30 minutes

INGREDIENTS:

- 3 cloves of garlic, chopped
- 3 tablespoons butter
- 3 cups whole corn kernels
- 8 ounces cream cheese
- 1 cup cheddar cheese
- 1 cup parmesan cheese
- 1 tablespoon salt
- ½ tablespoon black pepper
- ½ cup dry breadcrumbs
- 1 cup mozzarella cheese, grated
- 1 tablespoon thyme, minced

DIRECTIONS:

1. Fire the Traeger Grill to 350°F. Use desired wood pellets when cooking. Close the lid and preheat for 15 minutes.
2. In a large saucepan, sauté the garlic and butter for 2 minutes until fragrant. Add the corn, cheddar cheese, parmesan cheese, salt, and pepper. Heat until the corn is melted then pour into a baking dish.
3. In a small bowl, combine the breadcrumbs, mozzarella cheese, and thyme.
4. Spread the cheese and bread crumb mixture on top of the corn mixture.
5. Place the baking dish on the grill grate and cook for 25 minutes.
6. Allow to rest before removing from the mold.

NUTRITION INFORMATION:

Calories per serving: 523; Protein: 29.4g; Carbs: 34g; Fat: 31.2g Sugar: 10.8g

Grilled Corn on The Cob with Parmesan and Garlic

Serves: 6   **Cooking Time:** 30 minutes

INGREDIENTS:

- 4 tablespoons butter, melted
- 2 cloves of garlic, minced
- Salt and pepper to taste
- 8 corns, unhusked
- ½ cup parmesan cheese, grated
- 1 tablespoon parsley chopped

DIRECTIONS:

1. Fire the Traeger Grill to 450ºF. Use desired wood pellets when cooking. Close the lid and preheat for 15 minutes.
2. Place butter, garlic, salt, and pepper in a bowl and mix until well combined.
3. Peel the corn husk but do not detach the husk from the corn. Remove the silk. Brush the corn with the garlic butter mixture and close the husks.
4. Place the corn on the grill grate and cook for 30 minutes turning the corn every 5 minutes for even cooking.

NUTRITION INFORMATION:

Calories per serving: 272; Protein: 8.8g; Carbs: 38.5g; Fat: 12.3g Sugar: 6.6g

Grilled Asparagus with Wild Mushrooms

Serves: 4   **Cooking Time:** 10 minutes

INGREDIENTS:

- 2 bunches fresh asparagus, trimmed
- 4 cups wild mushrooms, sliced
- 1 large shallots, sliced into rings
- Extra virgin oil as needed
- 2 tablespoons butter, melted

DIRECTIONS:

1. Fire the Traeger Grill to 500°F. Use desired wood pellets when cooking. Close the lid and preheat for 15 minutes.
2. Place the asparagus, mushrooms, and shallots on a baking tray. Drizzle with oil and butter and season with salt and pepper to taste.
3. Place on a baking tray and cook for 10 minutes. Make sure to give the asparagus a good stir halfway through the cooking time for even browning.

NUTRITION INFORMATION:

Calories per serving: 218; Protein: 15.2g; Carbs: 26.6 g; Fat: 10g Sugar: 12.9g

Smoked 3-Bean Salad

Serves: 6   **Cooking Time:** 20 minutes

INGREDIENTS:

- 1 can Great Northern Beans, rinsed and drained
- 1 can Red Kidney Beans, rinsed and drained
- 1pound fresh green beans, trimmed
- 2 tablespoons olive oil
- Salt and pepper to taste
- 1 shallot, sliced thinly
- 2 tablespoons red wine vinegar
- 1 teaspoon Dijon mustard

DIRECTIONS:

1. Fire the Traeger Grill to 500°F. Use desired wood pellets when cooking. Close the lid and preheat for 15 minutes.
2. Place the beans in a sheet tray and drizzle with olive oil. Season with salt and pepper to taste.
3. Place in the grill and cook for 20 minutes. Make sure to shake the tray for even cooking.
4. Once cooked, remove the beans and place in a bowl. Allow to cool first.
5. Add the shallots and the rest of the ingredients. Season with more salt and pepper if desired. Toss to coat the beans with the seasoning.

NUTRITION INFORMATION:

Calories per serving: 179; Protein: 8.2 g; Carbs: 23.5g; Fat: 6.5g Sugar: 2.2g

Grilled Artichokes

Serves: 6   **Cooking Time:** 15 minutes

INGREDIENTS:

- 3 large artichokes, blanched and halved
- 3 + 3 tablespoons olive oil
- Salt and pepper to taste
- 1 cup mayonnaise
- 1 cup yogurt
- 2 tablespoons parsley, chopped
- 2 tablespoons capers
- Lemon juice to taste

DIRECTIONS:

1. Fire the Traeger Grill to 500°F. Use desired wood pellets when cooking. Close the lid and preheat for 15 minutes.
2. Brush the artichokes with 3 tablespoons of olive oil. Season with salt and pepper to taste.
3. Place on the grill grate and cook for 15 minutes.
4. Allow to cool before slicing.
5. Once cooled, slice the artichokes and place in a bowl.
6. In another bowl, mix together the mayonnaise, yogurt, parsley, capers, and lemon juice. Season with salt and pepper to taste. Mix until well-combined.
7. Pour sauce over the artichokes.
8. Toss to coat.

NUTRITION INFORMATION:

Calories per serving: 257; Protein: 6.7g; Carbs: 13.2 g; Fat: 20.9g Sugar: 3.7g

Grilled Scallions

Serves: 6   **Cooking Time:** 20 minutes

INGREDIENTS:

- 10 whole scallions, chopped
- ¼ cup olive oil
- Salt and pepper to taste
- 2 tablespoons rice vinegar
- 1 whole jalapeno, sliced into rings

DIRECTIONS:

1. Fire the Traeger Grill to 500°F. Use desired wood pellets when cooking. Close the lid and preheat for 15 minutes.
2. Place on a bowl all ingredients and toss to coat. Transfer to a parchment-lined baking tray.
3. Place on the grill grate and cook for 20 minutes or until the scallions char.

NUTRITION INFORMATION:

Calories per serving: 135; Protein: 2.2 g; Carbs: 9.7 g; Fat: 10.1g Sugar: 4.6g

Butter Braised Green Beans

Serves: 6　　**Cooking Time:** 20 minutes

INGREDIENTS:

- 24 ounces Green Beans, trimmed
- 8 tablespoons butter, melted
- Salt and pepper to taste

DIRECTIONS:

1. Fire the Traeger Grill to 500°F. Use desired wood pellets when cooking. Close the lid and preheat for 15 minutes.
2. Place all ingredients in a bowl and toss to coat the beans with the seasoning.
3. Place the seasoned beans in a sheet tray.
4. Cook in the grill for 20 minutes.

NUTRITION INFORMATION:

Calories per serving: 164; Protein: 1.6g; Carbs: 5.6 g; Fat: 15.8g Sugar: 1.3g

Smoked Baked Kale Chips

Serves: 4   **Cooking Time:** 30 minutes

INGREDIENTS:

- 2 bunches kale, stems removed
- Olive oil as needed
- Salt and pepper to taste

DIRECTIONS:

1. Fire the Traeger Grill to 350°F. Use desired wood pellets when cooking. Close the lid and preheat for 15 minutes.
2. Place all ingredients in a bowl and toss to coat the kale with oil.
3. Place on a baking tray and spread the leaves evenly on all surface.
4. Place in the grill and cook for 30 minutes or until the kale leaves become crispy.

NUTRITION INFORMATION:

Calories per serving: 206 ; Protein: 9.9g; Carbs: 21g; Fat: 12g Sugar: 0g

Smoked Pickles

Serves: 6   **Cooking Time:** 15 minutes

INGREDIENTS:

- 1-quart water
- ¼ cup sugar
- ½ quart white vinegar
- ½ cup salt
- ½ teaspoon peppercorns
- 1 ½ teaspoons celery seeds
- 1 ½ teaspoons coriander seeds
- 1 teaspoon mustard seeds
- 8 cloves of garlic, minced
- 1 bunch dill weed
- 12 small cucumbers

DIRECTIONS:

1. Place the water, sugar, vinegar, salt, and peppercorns in a saucepan. Bring to a boil over medium flame.
2. Transfer to a bowl and allow to cool. Add in the rest of the ingredients.
3. Allow the cucumber to soak in the brine for at least 3 days.
4. When ready to cook, fire the Traeger Grill to 500°F. Use desired wood pellets when cooking. Close the lid and preheat for 15 minutes.
5. Pat dry the cucumber with paper towel and place on the grill grate. Smoke for 15 minutes.

NUTRITION INFORMATION:

Calories per serving: 67; Protein: 2.4g; Carbs: 12.9g; Fat: 1.1g Sugar:8.5 g

Grilled Zucchini Squash

Serves: 6   **Cooking Time:** 10 minutes

INGREDIENTS:

- 3 medium zucchinis, sliced into ¼ inch thick lengthwise
- 2 tablespoons olive oil
- 1 tablespoon sherry vinegar
- 2 thyme leaves, pulled
- Salt and pepper to taste

DIRECTIONS:

1. Fire the Traeger Grill to 350ºF. Use desired wood pellets when cooking. Close the lid and preheat for 15 minutes.
2. Place zucchini in a bowl and all ingredients. Gently massage the zucchini slices to coat with the seasoning.
3. Place the zucchini on the grill grate and cook for 5 minutes on each side.

NUTRITION INFORMATION:

Calories per serving: 44; Protein: 0.3 g; Carbs: 0.9 g; Fat: 4g Sugar: 0.1g

Smoked Mushrooms

Serves: 6   **Cooking Time:** 10 minutes

INGREDIENTS:

- 4 cups baby portobello, whole and cleaned
- 1 tablespoon canola oil
- 1 teaspoon onion powder
- 1 teaspoon garlic powder
- Salt and pepper to taste

DIRECTIONS:

1. Place all ingredients in a bowl and toss to coat the mushrooms with the seasoning.
2. Fire the Traeger Grill to 350°F. Use desired wood pellets when cooking. Close the lid and preheat for 15 minutes.
3. Place mushrooms on the grill grate and smoke for 10 minutes. Make sure to flip the mushrooms halfway through the cooking time.
4. Remove from the grill and serve.

NUTRITION INFORMATION:

Calories per serving: 62; Protein: 5.2g; Carbs: 6.6g; Fat: 2.9g Sugar: 0.3g

Smoked Balsamic Potatoes and Carrots

☕ **Serves:** 6   🕐 **Cooking Time:** 10 minutes

INGREDIENTS:

- 2 large carrots, peeled and chopped roughly
- 2 large Yukon Gold potatoes, peeled and wedged
- 5 tablespoons olive oil
- 5 tablespoons balsamic vinegar
- Salt and pepper to taste

DIRECTIONS:

1. Fire the Traeger Grill to 400°F. Use desired wood pellets when cooking. Close the lid and preheat for 15 minutes.
2. Place all ingredients in a bowl and toss to coat the vegetables with the seasoning.
3. Place on a baking tray lined with foil.
4. Place on the grill grate and close the lid. Cook for 30 minutes.

NUTRITION INFORMATION:

Calories per serving: 219; Protein: 2.9g; Carbs: 27g; Fat: 11.4g Sugar:4.5 g

CPSIA information can be obtained
at www.ICGtesting.com
Printed in the USA
LVHW061409081020
668312LV00018B/151